YOUR KNOWLEDGE HAS VALUE

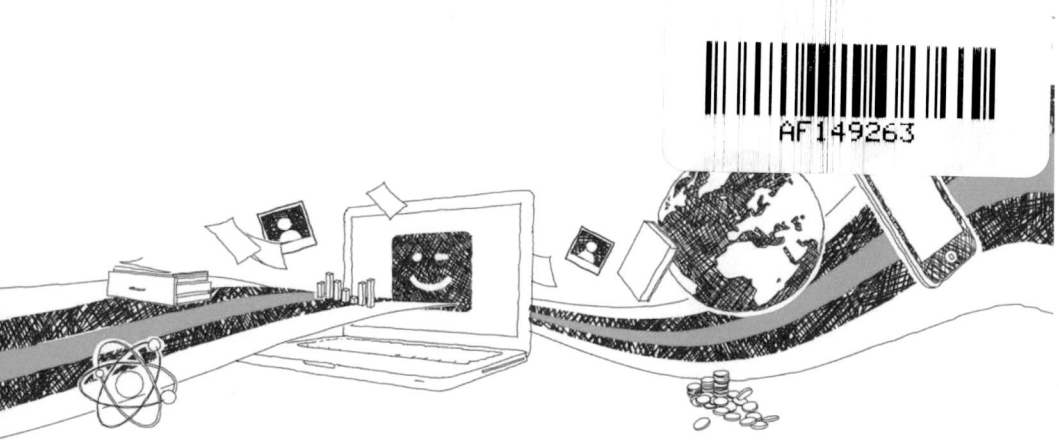
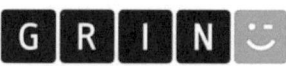

Bibliographic information published by the German National Library:

The German National Library lists this publication in the National Bibliography;
detailed bibliographic data are available on the Internet at http://dnb.dnb.de .

Imprint:

Copyright © 2017 GRIN Verlag, Open Publishing GmbH
Print and binding: Books on Demand GmbH, Norderstedt Germany
ISBN: 9783668574274

This book at GRIN:

http://www.grin.com/en/e-book/380745/primary-healthcare-practice-in-developing-
countries-a-case-study-of-india

Patrick Kimuyu

Primary Healthcare Practice in Developing Countries. A Case Study of India

GRIN Publishing

GRIN - Your knowledge has value

Since its foundation in 1998, GRIN has specialized in publishing academic texts by students, college teachers and other academics as e-book and printed book. The website www.grin.com is an ideal platform for presenting term papers, final papers, scientific essays, dissertations and specialist books.

Visit us on the internet:

http://www.grin.com/

http://www.facebook.com/grincom

http://www.twitter.com/grin_com

PRIMARY HEALTHCARE PRACTICE IN DEVELOPING COUNTRIES: CASE OF INDIA

Name: Patrick K. Kimuyu

Introduction

Assessing and improving primary healthcare has been an enormous challenge to the Healthcare Systems of developing countries around the globe. Therefore; lack of adequate healthcare services in most developing countries is believed to be the principal cause of short life-expectancy, owing to the high rates of mortality. In most developing countries, especially in Africa and Asia, policy makers and technical agencies do not seem to give primary healthcare high priority, and this is probably the reason as to why, healthcare standards in these countries have remained low, despite the immense effort by the International community. Moreover, most healthcare national programmes, which are initiated in developing countries to abase the public healthcare challenge, do not achieve remarkable success. Thomas (2009) claims, "The reasons for the failure of these national health programmes are multi-factorial. The most vital among these are the lackadaisical approach by the government officials involved in implementing the programmes" (p.1). On the other hand, population health issues seem to hinder significant development of most developing countries.

One of the most significant factors, which seem to have worsened the issue, is the rapid expansion of the populations within the developing countries. It has been found that, developing countries have the highest population growth rate compared to the wealthier nations such as the United Kingdom, Australia and the United States of America.

From an economic perspective, the disproportionate effect on the progress of developing countries can be attributed to the inadequate healthcare systems. Economic reports indicate that developing countries in dare need of healthcare systems are incurring enormous costs, owing to the burden of disease. Brink (2012) remarks, "A robust health system lies at the heart of building a country that has a healthy population, healthy society and healthy economy. The irony is that the countries that need those healthcare systems the most are paying the heaviest price" (par. 1). This phenomenon explains why healthcare influence development in developing countries. A healthy population plays a pivotal role in establishing a healthy economy of any country. However, it is worth noting that, the correlation between the progress of healthcare and national development follows diverse trends. For instance, change in demographic trends causes pressure on the existing public healthcare systems. Therefore, this research will give an overview on the concept of development and its links to health in India.

2

India's Demographic and Epidemiological Profile

India's demographic and epidemiological profiles explain the observed healthcare and national development issues. Currently, mortality rate has assumed an upward trend, and the public healthcare system is facing enormous disease burden. Medical reports indicate that demand for healthcare services have increased significantly; leading inaccessibility to essential medical services. Public healthcare facilities are also experiencing unprecedented pressure from the ever increasing population; thus, delivery of healthcare services in healthcare facilities has become compromised (Haub, 2009). Consequently, the Indian healthcare system has been characterized with low healthcare standards and healthcare resources utilization.

In general, demographic changes usually intersect with epidemiological patterns because; the two entities are inter-related. Therefore, India's health status is determined by the demographic and epidemiological trends. As such, it is worth evaluating the trends of these two factors to understand their impact on the national development, which is usually used as the principal determinant of the healthcare status. Moreover, it is also used to identify numerous economic inequalities that influence the health status of the population.

India's Demographic Profile

In a comprehensive review of India's demographic profile, population dynamics can be identified to enhance the prediction of India's economic growth. Demographic reports indicate that India is currently opening up numerous economic opportunities, owing to the progressive demographic changes, which have been occurring across the nation in the past decade. This has been so probably because; there is a significant decline of infant and child mortality, which has favoured population expansion. Bloom (2011) remarks, "Demographic change in India is opening up new economic opportunities. As in many countries, (including India), declining infant and child mortality helped to spark lower fertility; effectively resulting in a temporary baby boom" (p. 1).

Demographic reports indicate that India has been facing an enormous challenge of its population growth. Since 1951, the population of India recorded immense expansion, which created various demographic issues; thus, prompting the Government to design demographic approaches that were aimed at addressing developmental inequalities. By 1981, the population growth rate of India had increased by 24.7 % over a decade from 13.3 % growth rate recorded in 1951. However, India's population control measures were found to introduce significant improvement from 1971 onwards. For instance, the percentage population growth over decade decreased consistently from 24.8 %, in 1971 to 21.5 %, in 2001. Another impressive population growth factor, which seems to have increased economic potential of India, is the broadening of the working-age population. Moreover, the expansion of the urban population serves as an indicator of economic growth. Demographic reports indicate that India's urban population growth increased consistently from 17.3 %, in 1951 to 27.8 %, in 2001 (Kosh 2007).

India's Demographic Trends: Population Size and Growth, 1951-2001

Source: Kosh (2007)

According to the above data, appreciable demographic changes from 1971; a point at which population expansion started slowing down with an increase of the working-age population and urban population. From an analytical perspective, the observed demographic changes can be attributed to a decrease in infant and child mortality across India, leading an increase in the percentage of the working-age population. In addition, birth control programmes seem to have produced remarkable outcomes, and these trends have remained, more or less, the same up-to-date. Concisely, it appears true to state that India's opportunity to reap its demographic dividend has come because; its working-age population has increased remarkably to boost economic development, especially through expanding the country's labour force (Ingle & Suryawanshi 2011).

India's Demographic Transition and its Consequences for Development

India's demographic transition seems to have begun at a slow pace with gradual reduction in the average mortality rate. It is believed that the decline of famines and disease epidemics in the mid 1920s marked the country's demographic transition. Life expectancy of the Indian population recorded a significant increase with a substantial reduction of mortality rates and an increase in crude birth rates. As a result, India's population increased rapidly to reach a high mark of 336 million, by 1947 (Dyson 2008).

However, it is worth noting that the decrease in mortality rates in the subsequent decades was attributable to an array of factors. Some of the most fundamental factors included increased control of communicable diseases, immunization, and expansion of public healthcare facilities. Others included sustainable improvement of sanitation and increased spread of health education among within the population (Dyson 2008). It is also worth noting that there was a considerable delay in achieving a sustainable decline of mortality rates as there were delays in reaching a compensatory point, which was marked by a significant decline the average birth rates. However, recent demographic reports indicate that India has almost attained a state of equilibrium because; mortality rates have decreased significantly, whereas birth rates have remained at a sustainable level.

India's Epidemiological Profile

Currently, India's health profile appears to be impressive, owing to the transient improvements in a number of the core health related factors such as nutrition, health status of the Indian population and the socio-economic issues. In addition, eradication of chronic infectious diseases has contributed significantly to the observed epidemiological transition, although the burden of mortality seems to have shifted to noncommunicable diseases such as cancer, diabetes and heart failure (Armelagos & Harper 2010).

Burden of Disease

In general, burden of disease can be explained as trends of health challenges occasioned by the principal determinants and the risk factors of diseases and injuries. In epidemiological approaches, burden of disease is usually measured with regard to three core parameters: mortality, morbidity and disability, and the population's health status are also assessed in terms of these parameters.

In regard to the distribution of disease burden, India comes second in the Daily Adjusted Life Years (DALY) losses with a total of 268,953,000 deaths, in the global ranking.

Epidemiological reports indicate that Africa has the highest percentage of the global Daily Adjusted Life Years losses. In India, DALYs account for about 50% of the total burden of disease; whereas, noncommunicable diseases and injuries accounts for 33% and 17% respectively. Non-communicable diseases appear to be causing the highest mortality with infectious and parasitic infections accounting for a loss of 67,619 lives. Further epidemiological reports indicate that neuro-psychiatric disorders and cardiovascular diseases are among the Non communicable diseases with the highest contribution to the burden of disease. Among injuries, road accidents and falls accounts for a total loss of 19, 002 lives; thus, they are the largest contributors to disability burden (Gupte, Mutatkar & Ramachandran 2001).

Age and sex distribution patterns of the burden of disease can be evaluated through the use of malaria as an explicit example. In 1998, malaria mortality was found to be relatively higher among males than in females across all ages. The total number of malaria deaths in females was 1,654, roughly 36.95 compared to 2,827 deaths in males, which is equivalent to 63.1%. In regard to age-groups, individuals aged 15-54 years were the most affected, accounting to 56.1% followed by those aged >55 years accounting for 23.3%; whereas, infants and children aged below 14 years accounted for 20.6% of the total malaria deaths (Dash et.al. 2007).

India's Epidemiological Transition and its Consequences to Development

India's epidemiological transition appears to be influenced by an array of factors. Some of the most influential factors include the health status profile and community participation in health (Green 2007). Health profile involves maternal health, health financing, health services facilities, health policies and the nutritional status of the population. Infant and child health also play a crucial role in determining health profile.

In regard to nutrition, the net availability of food to the population appears to have increased by five-folds in the last 5 decades. Recent reports indicate that the production of food grains increased from 52.4 million tonnes, in the early 1950s to 203 million tonnes by 1998; although the net per capita (national agricultural output) of pulses seems to have dropped drastically from 60g, in 1951 to 36.3g, in 1993 (Gupte, Mutatkar & Ramachandran 2001).

On the other hand, infant and child health seem to have recorded a tremendous progress. Infant mortality rates have declined drastically from 222/1000 live births, in 1911 to 79/1000 live births, in 1998 (Gupte, Mutatkar & Ramachandran 2001). In addition, other health profile determinants such as maternal health, health services resources and health financing have progressed remarkably, owing to the efficient change of health policies by the Indian Government and the International health agencies.

However, it is worth noting that; despite the appreciable epidemiological transition, there are persistent challenges to primary healthcare, which appear to hinder absolute transition. For instance, malnutrition among women is one of the hindrances to appreciable epidemiological transition because; there is lack of efficient nutritional supplementation among adolescent girls and reproductive women. In addition, maternal and child health remain to be relatively low because; mortality rates among infants under the age of five years remain high. Moreover, sanitation and water supply has remained to be an enormous environmental issue because; 70% of the population do not have access to safe water supply and sanitation services in rural and urban centres (Gupte, Mutatkar & Ramachandran 2001). Therefore, such an unsafe environment is likely to cause healthcare problems, leading to the increase of the burden of disease.

India's Epidemiological Trends Compared to Australia

Epidemiological trends in developing countries are relatively different from those of developed countries. For instance, India faces its greatest burden of disease from infectious diseases and injuries. In contrast, Australia incurs the enormous burden of disease from noncommunicable diseases such as cancer, obesity and its related health problems. An outstanding example is the incidence rate of colorectal cancer. Australia is ranked among the developed countries with the highest incidence rates but, India falls in the lowest risk category (Boushey & Haggar 2009). In regard to infectious diseases, the recent epidemiological trends of TB in Australia and India give a distinctive feature on the situation. Prevalence rate of TB is relatively low in Australia compared to the ever increasing prevalence trends in India (Chadha 1997).

India's Development Prospects and Its Impact on Health

India appears to be on economic balance, owing to the current impact of demographic and epidemiological changes. Its economic prospects depend on the efficient acceleration of epidemiological and demographic transitions. Currently, there are three health-related and demographic potential threats to India's economic development. These are the effects of urbanization on health, population aging and population heterogeneity (Bloom 2011). The impact of urbanization of health is seemingly becoming a public healthcare problem because; chronic diseases have increased significantly since 1960. In 2005, chronic diseases accounted for 53% of the total deaths, in India. This was probably so because; the population living in urban areas has swollen rapidly from 18%, in 1960 to 30%, in 2008 (Bloom 2011).

On the other hand, the country is poised to reap its demographic dividends, owing to its population heterogeneity, in which the proportionality of the age structure favours labour productivity. However, efficient adjustments are required to improve the ratio of working-age to non-working-age populations across the country. The current demographic cycles have influenced India's economic status progressively. However, it is worth noting that the constructive synergy of its heterogeneity may create changes in the social and political landscapes because of economic inequalities among the population.

Another demographic threat to India's future economic prosperity is its population aging patterns. Today, the largest portion of India's population comprises of the working-age individuals. Demographic reports indicate that, only 16% accounts for the population aged >50 years. However, these age group is expected to increase rapidly by 2050 because the current cohort aged 15-50 years shall have crossed-over to the cohort aged >65 years. Therefore, dependency level may increase significantly, leading to economic retardation and decline in health status (Bloom 2011).

Conclusion

In a brief conclusion, primary healthcare in developing countries faces numerous challenges, owing to the current social and political features in the respective countries. It has been witnessed that, health status of the populations within developed countries is relatively high compared to that of developing countries. For instance, India has been facing numerous healthcare challenges; despite its impressive economic progress. This has been occasioned by the ignorance of policy makers who tend to undermine the impact of healthcare on the national GDP growth. As a result, sustainable epidemiological transition has never been realized; although the country has recorded a remarkable decline of mortality rates through improvement of healthcare resources. However, India's economy is expected to grow owing to the impact of its demographic transition. Nevertheless, appreciable economic development might never be realized; unless efficient healthcare policies are designed to avert the potential healthcare challenges. It is apparently true that, healthcare problems in developing countries can be eliminated through efficient public health measures.

References

Armelagos, G & Harper, K 2010, 'The Changing Disease-Scape in the Third Epidemiological Transition', *Int. J. Environ. Res. Public Health*, Vol. 7, pp. 675-697, Viewed 26 March 2013, via ijerph database, doi:10.3390/ijerph7020675.

Bloom, D 2011, *Population Dynamics in India and Implications for Economic Growth*, Viewed 18 Mar. 2013, <http://www.hsph.harvard.edu/pgda/WorkingPapers/2011/PGDA_WP_65.pdf>

Boushey, R & Haggar, F 2009, 'Colorectal Cancer Epidemiology: Incidence, Mortality, Survival, and Risk Factors', *Clin Colon Rectal Surg*, Vol. 22, no. 4, pp. 191–197, Viewed 22 Mar. 2013, < http://www.ncbi.nlm.nih.gov/pmc/articles/PMC2796096/>

Brink, B 2012, *Inadequate Health Systems Damage the Growth of Developing Nations, Media Release*, 8 Nov. 2012, Viewed 19 Mar. 2013, < http://www.guardian.co.uk/sustainable-business/poor-health-systems-damage-growth>

Chadha, V 1997, *Global Trends of Tuberculosis: An Epidemiological Review*, Viewed 22 Mar.2013, < http://openmed.nic.in/545/01/NLGLCH97.PDF>

Dash, P et.al, 2007, *Burden of Malaria in India: Retrospective and Prospective View*, Viewed 21 Mar. 2013, < http://www.ncbi.nlm.nih.gov/books/NBK1720/#>

Dyson, T 2008, *India's Demographic Transition and its Consequences for Development*, Viewed 20 Mar. 2013, < http://www.iegindia.org/timdysonlecture.pdf >

Green, A 2007, *An Introduction to Health Planning in Developing Health Systems, 3rd Edition*, Oxford, UK: Oxford University Press.

Gupte, M, Mutatkar, R & Ramachandran, V 2001, 'Epidemiological Profile of India: Historical and Contemporary Perspectives', *J. Biosci*, Vol. 26, No.4, pp. 437-463, Viewed 20 Mar. 2013, < http://www.ias.ac.in/jbiosci/nov2001/437.pdf>

Haub, C 2009, *India's Population Policy*, Viewed 28 Mar. 2013, < http://www.berlin-institut.org/online-handbookdemography/india.html >

Ingle, A & Suryawanshi, P 2011, *India's Demographic Dividend - Issues and Challenges*, Viewed 25 Mar. 2013, < http://www.trikal.org/ictbm11/pdf/Marketing/D1151-done.pdf>

Kosh, J 2007, *India's Population*, Viewed 17 Mar. 2013, < http://www.jsk.gov.in/indias_population.asp>

Thomas, V 2009, 'Healthcare in Developing Countries- Need for Finance, Education or Both?', *Calicut Medical Journal*, Vol. 7, No.1(e1), pp. 1-2, Viewed 22 Mar. 2013, <http://calicutmedicaljournal.org/2009/1/e1.pdf>

.

YOUR KNOWLEDGE HAS VALUE

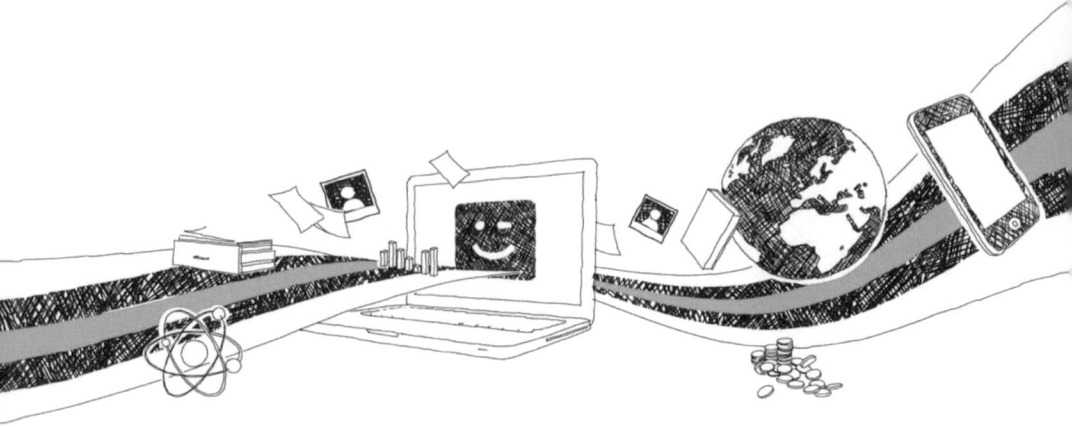

- We will publish your bachelor's and master's thesis, essays and papers

- Your own eBook and book - sold worldwide in all relevant shops

- Earn money with each sale

Upload your text at www.GRIN.com
and publish for free

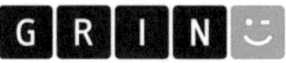